The Sabbath Season

Greg Smart

Parson's Porch Books

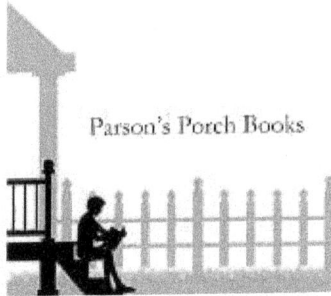

The Sabbath Season
ISBN: Softcover 978-1-960326-29-4
Copyright © 2023 by Greg Smart

Parson's Porch Books is an imprint of Parson's Porch & Company (PP&C) in Cleveland, Tennessee. PP&C is a self-funded charity which earns money by publishing books of noted authors, representing all genres. Its face and voice is **David Russell Tullock** (dtullock@parsonsporch.com).

Parson's Porch & Company *turns books into bread & milk* by sharing its profits with the poor.

www.parsonsporch.com

The Sabbath Season

Introduction

The medical staff was doing their pre-surgical routine, taking vitals and getting my medical information. The nurse was surprised to learn I was currently taking zero prescription medications.

"So, if it weren't for this," she said, "you'd be in really good health."

I replied sourly, "Ain't that the damn truth."

The, "this," was cancer.

At age 59, living an active life that included hiking, biking, soccer, and other forms of exercise, I'd suddenly been diagnosed with appendiceal cancer. The first surgery was to remove my appendix. Twelve days later, a second tumor was removed, along with half of my colon. Chemotherapy loomed on the horizon.

Until that diagnosis, the end of life was something I thought about only occasionally. Naturally, I dealt with death when it came to other families; that's what a pastor does. But my own final bow was something I assumed was at least thirty years in the future. And why not? My grandmother made it to 96, my father made it to 90, and my mother is still going strong. Sure, my grandfather died much earlier of lung cancer, but he smoked, so that didn't count. And my brother died of cancer at age 43, but that was a fluke.

This is what denial sounds like, by the way.

So, at age 59, I suddenly had to accept the reality that I might not make it to 62, much less the classic retirement age of 65.

But I wasn't alone. A church member had recently received a defibrillator. His grief began when the doctor told him the implant was only good for ten years. That's when this man was confronted by the reality of entering a new stage of life—a stage that comes with an expiration date.

This is a stage when you know your time is limited. We all know we're going to die, of course, but this is a stage of life when you realize that day is not far off. Sometimes it's a medical event that brings on this realization; other times it's reaching a certain age. Certainly, when you reach your eighties, you have to acknowledge there is only so much longer you can go on. Reaching 100 is a lot more common than it used to be but count how many centenarians you personally know. It's probably not a lot.

So, this new stage of life comes, and it hits hard. Along with grief comes plenty of self-reflection. And that reflection includes questions about faith. "Should I start apologizing to God now?" "Am I still faithful if I can no longer physically serve as an usher?" "What does God expect of me at this stage of my life?"

This is a book about life and faith in this closing stage. It grew out of a small-group study at Pikeville United Methodist, and it owes much to each of the participants.

In the opening chapter, we will begin to face the reality that we are but mortal. More than that, we'll face the reality that our time on earth is dwindling. Consequently, we'll begin to wrestle with the emotions such recognition unleashes.

Chapter Two looks at the loss of identity that comes with the last stage of aging. Who are you when you can no longer engage in the tasks and activities that have been a part of you for so long? In the final stages of life, there is the opportunity to simply accept oneself as God's beautiful child.

The third chapter introduces the concept of a Sabbath season. Just as retirement can be seen as a permanent vacation, our final years can be seen as a lasting season of Sabbath rest; a break from doing, and a time for simply being.

Chapter Four will examine some of the barriers to entering this Sabbath season. These are barriers we don't so much overcome as we move past by letting go.

Finally, the concluding chapter delves into the kind of healing that can take place even while we're dying. Such healing moves us fully into Sabbath, and into a peace like we've never known. This peace will carry us to our death and beyond, into that promised continuation of life.

What you read in these pages is hardly the authoritative word on the subject. You are free to disagree with me on any and all of it. But the hope is that this book will get you thinking about this subject and will bring you peace as eventide approaches.

Chapter One

It's the little things.

Like when a particular shirt or blouse becomes hard to button due to arthritis or neuropathy.

Or when you are forced to find a new position for putting on your socks.

Or maybe the stairs to your room have become the enemy.

Or all the things you can no longer remember.

And then there are the bigger moments.

A heart attack would certainly do it. So would a disabling car crash.

Or maybe it's a particular birthday and realizing you're now the same age as a mother or grandmother when she died.

Whatever brings it on, it's a moment when you are confronted by your own mortality. This is a realization that you're not going to live forever, and that your end may be closer than you think.

Watching our dog lumber around was one such moment. She was in her last weeks, and a regular dose of steroids was the only thing keeping her on her feet. As her strength faded, I realized that would be me one day, just holding on while playing out the string.

My cancer diagnosis accelerated the timeline from, "one day," to, "potentially soon."

Which is pretty much how it goes. Something will tip you off to your approaching end. That day may have moved substantially closer, or you may realize how close you've moved to that day. Whichever way it goes, you'll realize there just aren't that many days or years left.

That's a humbling moment, one that brings on many emotions, not the least of which is grief.

It can also bring on a panic. Suddenly you realize how much you still wanted to do or accomplish, and the clock is ever ticking, more audibly than before. Time to get moving… if only all those medical appointments weren't in the way.

More than anything, however, it's a moment of truth. It's accepting the reality that we will all die, and then changing the pronoun from "we" to "I," as in: "I will die someday."

Honestly, it takes a while to get used to saying that.

A good beginning, though, is to take an honest appraisal of your current situation. How's your health? How old are you? What's the life expectancy in your family? From there, you can do the math to see how many more years you might reasonably have. It might well be a sobering number, although it is only an estimate.

We were killing time on the golf course, waiting for the group ahead of us to move on. One of the guys mentioned his plans for when he turned 65. My comment was that he was planning awfully far ahead, and he replied, "That's only eight years away."

I had never done that math before, and the truth of it stunned me into silence. We were the same age, so it was eight years for me, too.

How old will you be in eight years? That's not even a decade. Yet, those kinds of numbers reflect the reality of being at a certain advanced age. And whether you get less or more years, it points unfailingly to your earthly destination. How you feel about that will set the stage for your remaining years.

There was a church that loved singing. The congregation made a joyful noise every time they got together. Their favorites all fit into the same category: In the Sweet, By and By; Beulah Land; When We All Get to Heaven; etc. They were all songs about passing from this life into the blessed next one, and how we should have no fear.

Yet, as I sat with the various families facing death, it became obvious those songs didn't reflect their true feelings. There was no peaceful embrace of death; these families fought death tooth and nail, throwing everything science could offer to stave it off.

There was also the large, suburban church where the music director once received hate mail for including All Creatures of Our God and King in Sunday worship. The words are from St. Francis of Assisi, and the sixth verse begins this way: "And thou, our sister, gentle death, waiting to hush our latest breath…"

That incensed one member enough to send in an angry letter. "Death is not our sister," began the letter, "death is the enemy!"

Maybe that's how you've always seen it, too. That's the way it's taught in many churches, based on the theological claim that death only exists because of that darn forbidden fruit in the Garden of Eden. If it hadn't been for that, goes this claim, we'd all live forever.

To the modern mind, which sounds like a nice fable. It's certainly not practical, and it raises a lot of questions. Yet, regardless of how you feel about what happened in Eden, death has been with us since the beginning. We have certainly had plenty of time to get used to the idea.

Despite that, many of us find death unsettling. We avoid the subject. We prefer celebrations of life over funeral services, because the latter seem too sad. It's also becoming more and more commonplace for people to attend visitations and skip the funeral, or for families to have no service at all. This was especially true during the COVID pandemic.

Then there's what goes on in the hospitals. Just watch how many families will walk out of the patient's room before even whispering the word, "death," or "dying." The doctors do it, too. They often don't want to acknowledge that reality. My experience has been that it's the nurses who are the most comfortable with the subject. If you want to know the truth of the situation, ask a nurse.

If you ever hope to be comfortable with the subject, you have to face it. If you want to make peace with death, then you have to talk about it. The same is true for your family. While I managed to make peace with the fact that my cancer could end my life rather soon, no one else in the family wanted to acknowledge that or even mention it.

If you're not sure how your family feels about the subject, here's a simple experiment: prepare an advance directive/living will, then schedule a family meeting to discuss your wishes. For most families this will be a time of uneasy squirming and last-minute excuses. It certainly won't be like gathering for the holidays. The reality of death, especially death coming for a loved one, is something most people just don't want to acknowledge.

The general pattern is that the dying person knows he or she is dying. Meanwhile, everyone else is tiptoeing around the subject, avoiding it with the same effort one might avoid a landmine.

That's not a healthy way to approach death. That kind of avoidance prevents the peace we can have at eventide; the peace that is possible in our last days, weeks, months, or years.

If that's the kind of peace you crave, please keep reading. For now, though, if you are in a position to know your days are dwindling, take seriously this next suggestion.

Simply write down the feelings you're experiencing. Be as specific as possible. There are a lot of things we can lump under grief or anger; maybe what you're more specifically feeling is dismay, or a loss of direction, or a sense of unfairness about it all. There are plenty of websites that have downloadable feelings charts to help with this task.

The reason for exploring these emotions is that, when we can name what we're feeling, we're then in a much better place to deal with it. Think of it as a diagnosis. With the feeling identified, treatment can begin. We realize which feelings are natural in such a circumstance, and which might indicate a deeper issue. Those deeper issues will require additional work, perhaps even outside aid. The normal feelings are ones we have to welcome in, rather than resist. We just have to go through them, so we can come out on the other side as a whole person.

Through this process, we move towards acceptance of the situation. And once you've accepted the dwindling time for what it is, then

you're in a position of readiness for wholeness
and peace.

Chapter Two

"If you go to Atlanta, the first question people ask you is, "What's your business?" In Macon they ask, "Where do you go to church?" In Augusta they ask your grandmother's maiden name. But in Savannah the first question people ask you is, "What would you like to drink?"

John Berendt, *Midnight in the Garden of Good and Evil.*

You are not your job.

Yet, many people's whole identity is built around what they do for a living. This is captured in the extremely common conversation opener: "What do you do?" After a while, it's easy to see one's self as a doctor, teacher, engineer, etc. The problem comes when one retires. Once you're no longer a doctor, what are you?

This is precisely why some people don't retire. Bear Bryant apparently couldn't live as a retired football coach. He died of heart failure four weeks after coaching his last game. Though his retirement was clouded in scandal, Joe Paterno suffered the same fate. He died of lung cancer roughly a month after his last game as coach.

Some will tell you they simply love the job too much to ever retire. Betty White was still a working actress when she died less than a month shy of turning 100.

Then there are those who feel their jobs are just too important to leave, and those who have jobs that are for life. Ruth Bader Ginsburg stayed on as a Supreme Court Justice until her death at age 87. Queen Elizabeth remained queen until her death. But then there is Pope Benedict XVI, who became only the second pope (and the first in 600 years) to retire, citing a lack of strength in mind and body. He was 83 at the time.

If you live long enough, you will experience a weakened mind and/or body. Even if you're young, disease can sap your vitality and mental acuity. For many people, this is what leads to a loss of identity. Maybe this decrease in motor and cognitive function forces you to retire. Maybe you have to step back from any volunteer work or other activities that have filled your time. Maybe this restricted version of your body doesn't fit in with your self-image.

Whichever might be the case, the end result is a loss of identity. You're no longer the technician, nurse, teacher, tradesman, volunteer, repairman, supermom, or strapping young man you used to be. And that's just the loss of a professional identity.

It can also be a crushing blow to have to step back from a role at the church. It's not unusual to see elderly ushers hobbling down the aisle, because to give up that area of service would be too much. That person may have been an usher for decades. He (typically) may not know how to simply sit in worship. He may have trained multiple generations of ushers. To admit to being physically unable to do the task would be to have one foot in the grave.

The same could be said of servants within the altar guild, the church office, the choir, Sunday school teachers, etc. Yes, there's a loss of prestige, respect, and even power when stepping down from such positions, but the feeling that leaves you feeling lost is that loss of identity. Who are you within the church when you are no longer the head usher or the one who counts the offering?

The choir director and pianist at one church had come to the point where it was time to step down. She was in the early stages of dementia, and it was coming out in multiple ways. She was having trouble reading music, she was forgetting explicit instructions during worship, and she was breaking down emotionally during rehearsals. To continue in that role wasn't good for the church, and it wasn't good for her. The stress was actually exacerbating her condition. When the church came to her and her husband with the decision, it wasn't received well. Yet, the most heart-broking moment came when the husband said, "Leading the choir is who she is."

There's also a loss of identity when you out-live your family and friends. Many a person from a large family feels lost when realizing she is the last one standing. Who are you in the family when there are no more siblings to pick up the phone?

Then there's the loss of human connection when your deteriorating mobility and motor skills restrict you to the house. As you venture out less and less often, your social circle shrinks dramatically. This is also a loss of identity. No longer are you the funny one, the leader, the organizer, or the one in which your friends confide. The world seems to be going on without you as you slowly fade away.

All of this is plenty to deal with as it is, then you throw in the realization that this physical and mental diminishment will eventually lead to death.

This is a crisis, and you begin to see yourself as a withered body, just living out the string. In short, you begin to feel useless. This feeling can be so strong that it's common to wonder what point there is to go on living at all.

That may sound harsh, but it's a sentiment that has been expressed by many a church member who suddenly finds him or herself homebound, incapacitated, or on the sidelines. Even John Wesley had that fear. He confided in his journal on December 22, 1763: "Lord, let me not live to be useless!" He was only 60 at the time, yet that is the cry of a man whose whole identity was bound up in his service to God; so much so, that he preferred death to the thought of losing that identity. It's no wonder so many in this position are prescribed anti-depressant and anti-anxiety medication.

However, our identity is in God, not in our ability to serve others. This is the God who names us and gives us new names. This is the God who changed Abram to Abraham and Sarai to Sarah. This is the God who changed Saul to Paul, and Simon to Peter. These are names that reflect our truest identity, the identity we were given when God made us. We never were our jobs, because we have always been God's.

Furthermore, we have always been precious to God. Consider Psalm 139:13-16. God has known you from your very beginning.

Consider also Luke 3:21-22. I personally believe the words spoken to Jesus at his baptism also apply to us; that these were God's words to you at your baptism. You also are God's beloved child. God is well-pleased with you.

You may immediately want to point to the obvious differences between Jesus and yourself. You, of course, are not the Messiah, much less given sight to the blind or raised anyone from the dead. That is true enough. But those words from heaven were spoken before Jesus did any of those things. They are words of unconditional love; the feelings of a parent for a child. That child is loved just because. And that undercurrent of love survives even the nastiest of storms.

God loves you the same way. God loved you before you were born. God loved you before you received your first report card in school. God loved you before you ever held a job. Your relationship with God was never performance-based. Why should it be now? You are loved just as you have always been loved.

In Psalm 71:9, the psalmist cries out: "Do not cast me off in the time of old age; do not forsake me when my strength is spent." This is a feeling to which we can relate. But hear the assurance in Isaiah 49:15: "Can a woman forget her nursing child, or show no compassion for the child of her womb? Even these may forget, yet I will not forget you."

You were God's before you were born. You will be God's after your death. Yet, the greater assurance is that you are loved by God just as you are; for better, for worse; for richer, for poorer; in sickness and in health; to love and to cherish.

Now that you know that, now that you have this assurance of being God's beloved, we turn to the big questions. What does faith look like when light is fading? How do you follow Jesus when you can no longer get out of bed? What are you to do with your remaining days when you can no longer serve God as before?

We begin to answer that in the next chapter.

Chapter Three

He was just sitting there, quietly gazing upon the world God had made.

He was no longer the man he had once been; a man who could build anything, a man who had traveled the world, a man who had taken on adventures in the service of his Lord.

Parkinson's Disease had slowed him down. He still loved puttering around in his workshop, but tasks that used to take minutes now took hours. Although his mind was still facile, he now had trouble making the words come. He also drooled a little. Discreetly, he carried a handkerchief to dab away the moisture.

Still, he was a portrait of a man at peace. Sitting there on the bench, looking serenely at the birds, the clouds, and the gently blowing leaves, he was perfectly filling the role God had given him.

Think of how you would define Sabbath. Hundreds of books have been written on the subject, and from these rich resources we get definitions like: a day dedicated to the Lord; a cessation of work; a day of rest; a breaking of patterns; complete trust in God; even celebration.

Yet, no matter the definition, we tend to view Sabbath as a temporary period. The weekly Sabbath, of course, is a day. We might extend the length if we consider a vacation to be a Sabbath period. Then there's the professional sabbatical, which might last a few months to a year. All of these, however, refer to a temporal event through which we pass. We enter Sabbath, we experience Sabbath, and when it is over we go back to our regularly scheduled programming.

Then there's the man on the bench. Pete was his name. And Pete had entered Sabbath season.

This is one of those times when you are free to disagree, but I believe we enter a Sabbath season in the closing stages of life. When the body, when the mind, can no longer do the work we've been given, that's when we begin a lasting Sabbath. In that season, we enjoy all the ways Sabbath has been defined.

Think of those final years, months, days as a season dedicated to the Lord. This could look like Judith. She is 95 years old, and her joy is attending worship when she is able. When she can't, she sits looking out her picture window, drinking in the wonders of creation. Surrounding her are her Bible and numerous books of prayers and devotions. On her face is a constant smile. On her lips is praise for God. Her days of teaching Sunday school and serving on committees are behind her. She is in a Sabbath season, and God is pleased.

Think of Sabbath as a cessation of work. Unless you die suddenly, the day will come when you can no longer toil at a profession or tirelessly volunteer within community or church. While we may lament having to move from the playing field to the bleachers, God does not.

When God calls Jeremiah to be a prophet, Jeremiah quickly says, "I do not know how to speak; I am too young." God's equally quick response is, "Do not say, 'I am too young,' …for I am with you…" (Jer. 1:6-8) What's entertaining about this exchange is Jeremiah's assumption. He seems to think God has no idea how old Jeremiah is. It's almost as if God must have made some mistake; that God had shown up at the wrong address. We know better, of course. God knew exactly whom he was calling.

The same thing is true when we find ourselves weakened in our final stages. God is not surprised by our physical state. God is not caught off guard by our diminished mental faculties. God knows exactly what's going on with us. This decrease in ability is the natural path humans travel. It's only when life is cut short that we don't experience this diminishment. And if this is the natural path for God's beloved children, don't you think God has a plan for that? Sabbath season is that plan.

A clergy colleague is in the first stages of dementia. This is a man who has served churches in several regions of the country. He's even planted a few. When he no longer had the energy to pastor a church, he found a way to continue serving God: he began duty as a cruise ship chaplain. Now, with his memory deserting him, he's found it's time to step back from the pulpit. Rather than bemoaning his fate, he has decided to embrace this season of his life. He has taken a few final trips to places he'd always wanted to see, and he is simply enjoying his days with family and friends. The end of his working days has allowed him to find the joy in his Sabbath season.

The end of work, and the end of volunteer labor, are both a breaking of patterns. The old rhythms of life are over, and a new dance begins. This was stated clearly by a retiring physician. He rejoiced that he no longer had to rise daily to the blaring of the alarm clock. Actually, he vowed to never use one again.

With this new freedom from work schedules and old responsibilities, you are now free to simply live. Life is a gift, and the breaking of patterns gives you time to enjoy that gift. Spend time with the people you most enjoy. Do the things that put a smile on your face. There are no more demands on you, no more expectations. Sabbath season is a time to feel the warmth of God's love.

What makes all this possible is another way of understanding Sabbath: as a time of putting your trust fully in God.

One of the most important lessons I learned in my early work life was that I was not indispensable. That seems like a strange thing to embrace. We all want to feel important, at least to someone. Yet, to realize that the world would not come crashing down if I couldn't make it in to the office was very freeing. It meant that I could go on vacation without fretting over what was happening without me. The real lesson was that I could trust my co-workers to handle whatever came up while I was gone, just as I could pick up the slack when they were absent.

In the same way, Sabbath is putting complete trust in God. Chick-fil-a is a good example of this. The fast food giant is famously closed on Sundays. Management trusts that, despite the gobs of money they're leaving on the table, they will have enough. Of course, when you're making millions, that's an easy trust.

Still, the principle applies. To not go into the office on Sunday is to trust that God will not let you starve just because you decided to rest or to spend that day with family. And in the Sabbath season of life, we are trusting that we are in God's hands. We trust that God will not forsake us; that God will be there in our death, just as God was there in our birth. That's a critical notion. The ultimate question of faith is not, "Do we trust God with our life," it's, "Do we trust God with our death?" When we accept that death is part of life, we open the door to trusting God.

It also turns out that such trust opens our eyes to new truths. In his book, Sacred Fire, Ronald Rolheiser raises an intriguing idea: that we are not useless when our limbs and minds no longer function. Noting that the word patient and passive come from the same Latin word,

Rolheiser makes an interesting point: a patient is passive; a patient receives care from others. In that role of patient, the receiver is granting a gift to the one providing the care, for the giver is learning how to give; the giver is learning how to care in a brand new way.

This is true whether the caregiver is a professional or a member of the family. Doctors and nurses learn how to interact with people in new ways during the course of their work. They also learn to do things they may have thought they would never do. There's no place for the squeamish when inserting a catheter.

As for family, my relationship with my oldest son was changed forever when he spent three weeks helping out during my chemotherapy. He was considerate and attentive, and may have shown the most important trait of a caregiver: instead of making assumptions, he asked what was needed or desired. Armed with that information, he began to anticipate my needs. As a result, I love that boy more than ever, and I really came to trust him during those weeks.

When we come to have that same kind of trust in the Lord, when we know God is there for us, when trust defines our relationship with our

Creator, then we can rest. This is another area where we might have to adjust our thinking.

Typically, we think of rest as what we do to recharge our batteries, to rejuvenate and be ready for the next round. It's like the rest you might take after a steep climb on a hike. You need time to catch your breath, before resuming the hike. That's certainly how we think of the rest that comes with the weekly Sabbath.

The season of life we're talking about, however, is lasting rest. This Sabbath will carry us into the continuation of life. And perhaps we do need to rest before the glorious what's next. Yet, it might be more helpful to think of this rest as the kind of rest you get after a good day's work. With the labor finished, you can sit on the porch, satisfied and free to enjoy the evening breeze. There are no more deadlines, no more work to be done, there is nothing to do but enjoy the life you've been given.

Actually, there is one thing more that needs to be done: celebrate. In addition to all the other ways Sabbath can be defined, Sabbath is also a celebration of all God has provided, and of all the ways God has been present in your life. That doesn't mean you have to have loud music or a wild party. You can celebrate internally, praising God for all the gifts you have received.

Pete had a deep connection to nature. He'd even built a frog pond at his home. So, it was no surprise that day to find him gazing at what God had built. The surprise was how serene he was. He had entered Sabbath season, and he was content.

The scene was the same the last time I saw him alive. Pete could no longer speak, but when he had the strength he wanted to sit in a chair gazing out at his backyard, a yard that gave way to a wooded area. That's what I found him doing. He was at peace seeing Creation at its daily best: squirrels scurrying about; birds flitting from branch to branch; the ground awash in leaves; all in a sun-dappled tableau. In his peace and contentment, Pete was teaching those who visited him about Sabbath season.

Chapter Four

It was a hot summer day. There are no other kind in Florida. It was even hotter up on the roof, where a group of us from the church were putting a new roof onto the building of a sister congregation. All that was left to do was to finish the shingles.

That was the work in which I was engaged. It was work I enjoyed. Because of the heat, I was due for a mandatory water break, but I wanted to get to a good stopping point first. In my mind, that meant finishing the current line. When I reached the end, however, I realized I already had the chalk marked out for the next line, so I went ahead and started that line of shingles.

With the sun beating down, I told myself I'd get off the roof for a break as soon as I finished this new line. I was serious this time, since I could feel what the heat was doing to me. But, gosh, I already had the shingles at hand. Putting them on wouldn't take long. Actually, I had a whole bag of shingles there. I should probably put them all on before the tar started to melt. I could hold out while I nailed down a few more shingles. I could even start yet another new line. It wouldn't take that long.

I was no longer sweating at that point. I was dehydrated. But those shingles had to go on that roof. I finally stopped when I realized what was happening.

The heat had gotten to me. I wasn't thinking straight. I was actually becoming frantic about the work; thinking I had to get those shingles up, or they wouldn't get done.

That was nonsense, of course. We had plenty of guys to do the work, and most of them were a lot more skilled than I was. I had simply gotten to a point where I couldn't let go. Yet, letting go is necessary before we can enter Sabbath.

Sabbath season awaits, but entering it is not always easy. Much of what makes us human becomes the very barrier that keeps us from going where God is beckoning. Our drive and ambition, the desire to help others, the pride in all we have accomplished and acquired, our responsibilities, our deeply felt and deeply precious relationships; all of these can keep us clinging to life. The thought of letting go seems worse than death; or perhaps it is death. For many of us, letting go seems like the same thing as pulling the plug on our own lives. It feels like giving up, like quitting. And we're not quitters.

What is necessary for letting go is to put our trust in God. This is more than trusting that God will catch you; this is trusting that you still matter to God even when you let go of all that has made up the person you believe yourself to be. This is trusting that you matter to God just because your heart beats and your lungs draw breath. And of course you matter, because God gave you that heart and put that breath within you. You matter to God simply because you have life.

The first act of trust, then, is to let go and let God. This is where the 12-step programs have it right. Stop trying to control everything, and let God be in charge. This will mean letting go of some ways that have served you well.

For starters, you'll be letting go of thinking you have to do everything yourself. That was the mistake I was making on the roof. That roof was going to get done whether or not I ever nailed down another shingle. There were other people who could handle the job, just as there will be other people to do the job once you retire.

You'll also have to let go of thinking the job has to be done your way, whether it's a paid or volunteer job. Other people actually have good ideas. Believe it or not, their way of doing things works just as well as yours. They can solve problems, too. Sometimes, they'll solve problems you can't. They might even find a more efficient way to get a task done. To think your way is the only way, or the absolute best way, is pretty arrogant.

Along with letting go of your way, it's also necessary to let go of thinking a task has to be done right now. One thing I learned from working in several different industries, is that most deadlines are false. Deadlines are helpful; no argument there. But all is not lost if a deadline is not met.

Working at an advertising agency, there was a project on which unforeseen delays caused us to miss several hard deadlines. Every single time, we realized there was another way we could still deliver the work. We finally got everything done, and one of the employees personally drove to the client two hours away, to hand-deliver the finished project.

It also comes as a shock to many people to realize dirty dishes don't come with a deadline. Sometimes more important things come up. At those times, the dishes can wait. Even the IRS will grant an extension. So, let go of the idea that some given task has to be done right then and there. Such thinking will only lead to anxiety. And anxiety is a barrier to Sabbath.

The last thought to let go of is that a thing has to be done at all. It will be a shame if the company you built over 50 years goes out of business after you sell it, but it won't be the end of the world. For all those years, your company provided needed goods or services to your customers. That was a gift to all those people, a gift you made possible. But businesses have life cycles, too. They're born, and they die.

The same goes with personal tasks. That last project you wanted to complete? The world will keep turning if you don't get to it. Just think of all the authors and composers who didn't get to finish their last offering. Franz Schubert's famous Unfinished Symphony comes to mind. For whatever reason, he never got around to finishing it. Maybe the finished product would have been his best work, but it really doesn't matter; the world was still enriched by his previous efforts.

So, let go of thinking, "I have to do it." Let go of thinking, "It has to be done my way." Let go of thinking, "It has to be done now." And let go of thinking, "It has to be done." Instead, let go and let God.

This does not mean you have to stop doing the things you enjoy. It might mean, however, you have to find a new way to do those things, or that you stop doing them to earn your keep. And it definitely means stop being frantic about those activities.

Since recovering from cancer treatment, I've been playing soccer in an adult league. My team is not going to win any championships, and I'm not exactly setting the world on fire. There was a point in my life that would have driven me nuts. Back then, I had to win. Now? I'm thrilled to be able to play at my age. And being in a league means I can count on playing once a week, with a group of people I enjoy. I wouldn't turn down a few more wins, but I don't need them. Just being in a competitive game is win enough.

Letting go of that need brings freedom. I'm free to enjoy seeing a full moon over the pitch. I'm free to admire the skills of other players. I'm free to celebrate a struggling player finally scoring a goal. You'll find similar enjoyment once you let go of the frantic struggle to get ahead, to achieve, to excel, to produce. You'll also find the freedom to enter Sabbath. Yet, there are a few more things that need to be released before that final freedom comes.

You can start by letting go of worries. There was a man in his eighties who was suffering from several ailments. He confided that he was ready to pass on, ready to rest, ready to rejoin his deceased wife. It was a beautiful moment, and it gave this man peace to say it out loud. After a moment of holy silence, the man then blurted out, "But I'm so mad about China."

He went on to say he hated leaving his children to live in a world colored by the global issues between the U.S. and China. The feeling was understandable, but what was this man going to do about that? Shouting at the TV wasn't going to change anything. And at his age, combined with his health issues, shouting was about all he could do.

Is that how he really wanted to go to his grave? That man's worry over China was a barrier to Sabbath. He had voiced his readiness, his acceptance of his situation, but that needless worry was keeping him from being truly at peace. Whatever worries still burden you, release them. Turn them over to God. There's no need for you to carry them anymore.

You will also need to release your former identities. This was discussed in an earlier chapter, yet it's one of the most difficult things to do.

On the show Ted Lasso, legendary player Roy Kent was facing retirement. He knew he was no longer the player he was before, plus he had suffered a major injury, but he was fearful of losing his identity. Football was all he had known. It was only when his adoring niece said she loved him because he's a great uncle that he was able to retire. Of course, that niece is just like God in that instance. God loves us in every season of our lives, even when there's no longer a nameplate on an office door.

Or consider the man who retired to his quaint hometown. He immediately became the president of the local chamber of commerce, and took on chairmanship of a church committee. Then, a heart episode resulted in a much-need realization. The man confessed that all his life he had gravitated to positions of leadership; that he could never just serve on a board or committee, he had to lead it. That recognition led him to relinquish his leadership positions so that he could find the beauty in simply serving. He also found a beauty in himself, once his identity was no longer tied up in being a leader.

The last thing to release would be some deeply felt responsibilities. These will vary from person to person, but they include professional and volunteer responsibilities, household responsibilities, and familial responsibilities.

Look at the story of Dorcas in Acts 8:36-43. As Dorcas lay lifeless in that upper chamber, all kinds of people had gathered to grieve. They were weeping and showing the garments this saintly woman had made for them. With her gone, who would do that important work for the poor?

From a certain perspective, it's a shame that Paul, through the Holy Spirit, restored her life. Returned from the dead, Dorcas could resume her work. Crisis averted. However, it was also an opportunity removed. Had Dorcas stayed dead, maybe someone who had been greatly moved by Dorcas' work would have picked up the mantle. Maybe this person would have even expanded the ministry, bringing in all kinds of new people who would be blessed by giving out blessings. As long as you tightly grip your responsibilities, someone else will not discover their own gifts.

There was an elderly man who headed up a local food bank. As is often the case, the local food bank was much bigger than most people would suspect. It had a six-figure annual budget, and was feeding hundreds of people each month. The president was doing a fine job of running this ministry. He was also quite qualified, having served under General Patton during WWII.

However, the man was nearing 90, and his physical powers were visibly eroding. He was also grieving the passing of his wife. With all of that going on, he decided it was time to step down and let someone else run the food bank.

This would have been an important step in this man's life, had he actually followed through. Five months later, he was still the president, still making all the decisions, and still there every time the doors of the food bank were opened. He couldn't let go. Partly that was because he was trying to fill the void that comes with being a widower. Partly that was because he didn't think anyone else could do the job as well as he could; he certainly found none of the candidates for the role to be a suitable replacement. And partly it was because he was afraid of what would happen to him if he stopped doing that work.

Contrast that with the food bank in another town. The pastors of the ministerial association ran it, but they had long wanted to relinquish that responsibility. After years of voicing that desire, they finally decided to just do it. They brought together people from their respective congregations to form a leadership board, then handed them the keys. Within three years that food bank had situated itself in a better location, established two satellite locations, and had increased the number of people served by five hundred percent.

The fears we have of relinquishing our responsibilities are often completely unfounded. Worse, we sometimes do more harm by holding on than the good we imagine we're doing.

There are situations in which you can make a plan of succession. If that fits your setting, make a plan, then follow through. If a succession plan is not doable in your case, you may just have to step down. If the work is worth continuing, someone will step up. Or maybe it's time for the work to end. Either way, let go and trust God with the rest.

The responsibility that holds so many people captive is the responsibility they feel to family. This feeling is especially keen when minor children are still in the house. Cancer and other illnesses play a cruel game with young families. Then there are the older parents concerned about a child that never seemed to get life on track. Or the parents who leave behind a special needs child. These and other situations leave folks clinging to their last days, filling their hearts and minds with anguish and anxiety.

If this is a responsibility with which you struggle, get ready for some blunt advice: face the reality of your situation and take the necessary steps for those who will survive you. For starters, make out a will. There's really no excuse for putting off this step any longer. While you're at it, make sure the beneficiaries of your insurance and your other accounts are who you want them to be.

It would also be wise to prepare an advance directive; what was formerly known as a living will. This should be a clear statement of what you want and do not want for medical care, including hospice. Think now about what kind of care you want in case you are unresponsive. Do you want to be on a ventilator? Do you want a feeding tube? Do you want "heroic measures" if you were to flatline? Making such decisions now can save your family untold amounts of fretting, as well as some animosity.

Carl died. He quit breathing. He was turning blue. Medical personnel were able to revive him, and he was then placed in ICU. His three sons gathered around him, as they should have at that important time. The problem was that Carl had communicated his wishes to only one of those sons, the oldest. The other sons, not being privy to those wishes, and reacting purely out of their emotions, did not believe their older brother. So, while Carl had expressed no wish to be kept alive artificially, the ensuing disagreement between his sons kept the machines going for another 30 days; thirty days in which Carl was unconscious, just a prone body lying in a hospital bed. He even died a second time, only to be revived once more. Then came word that the brothers had thrown a few punches at each other and had to be escorted out of the hospital.

All of that could have been avoided had Carl only communicated his wishes to his family. Unfortunately, Carl had not written anything down; he simply discussed it one night with the son who was there. What a gift, however, Carl could have given his family had he prepared a written advance directive. Then his sons could have come together in grief, rather than being torn apart by their own opinions as to what was best.

It's also a great idea to prearrange your funeral. This will take an enormous burden off your family, both financially and emotionally. Grieving children make lousy decisions. Guilty children make expensive decisions. So, go ahead and choose your own casket or opt for cremation. Pre-pay it if you can. Most funeral homes have a guide that will help you pick your burial site, the funeral location, clergy preference, even the music you want.

Once you have made these decisions and taken care of the necessary documents, inform your children and other survivors of your wishes, clearly answering any questions that come up. You'll also want to make sure your survivors can find those documents, whether they're in a desk drawer, safety deposit box, or filed with an attorney. And don't bother trying to spare anyone's feelings in that meeting. Your survivors are going to have feelings; that's unavoidable. But those feelings are theirs to deal with, not yours. Your job is to take care of business.

And if you want to go the extra mile, start getting rid of your stuff. That is a true gift to your children and your spouse. My uncle was brilliant when the time came. He was downsizing and had a houseful of furniture he wouldn't need. There were plenty of other items, as well, some of which had been in the family for decades. Giving his children plenty of notice, this man announced a deadline. Anything they hadn't claimed by that day would go into an estate sale. The brilliance of this was that it didn't put an unreasonable burden on the children. They had a fair chance to get anything they wanted, with no responsibility to dispose of the rest.

You are the person best suited to handle old photographs and keepsakes. The same is true of paperwork you've kept for decades. Get rid of it and spare your children or spouse the work.

As for what becomes of your children after you pass, let go and let God. If your children are baptized, they belong to God already. And just like baby birds, they have to learn to fly sometime. If they haven't done so by now, they need a different teacher.

In the category of unlikely sources for a book on Sabbath season, Lee Child wrote something profound in one of his Jack Reacher tales. In *The Enemy*, Reacher's mother said your children's lives are like going into a movie theater knowing you won't get to see the ending; you just don't know when you have to leave.

Celebrate who your children are, not who you wish they were. Make your preparations, and then the rest is up to them. This is the way it has been since the beginning.

These are the things that need to be released, and letting go is the necessary step. You can't take your money or your stuff with you, nor can you take your worries. Entrust it all to God once you've done all you can do. Then you can enter the blessed lasting season of Sabbath.

Chapter Five

Maybe you've been there. Maybe you've heard the doctor say there is no cure, or that there's nothing more that can be done.

If so, you remember what came next: a flood of emotions. Your heart sank into your stomach, and the tears began to fall. As you grappled with the news, you grappled also with a range of feelings, the biggest of which was grief.

No matter who was the subject of the news, the same things were grieved. You grieved for yourself, feeling the devastating truth in the depths of your soul. You grieved the relationships that would end, already dreading the good-byes. Really, you grieved all that would be lost. If it was a spouse or a sibling, you grieved the phone conversations you would no longer have, and the emptiness on holidays and other special occasions. If you were the one who learned your days were dwindling, you grieved the sunsets and the seasons, driving on the open road, watching your favorite team, and all the other things that make living such a joy.

Dave had gotten to a point where he could no longer eat. His sustenance came from a feeding tube. He was asked if he missed eating. His reply was that he missed, not the cheeseburger itself, but the idea of a cheeseburger. We remember those wonderful sensations, and we grieve their passing.

The grief that comes with hearing the word "terminal" is natural. It can also be a barrier to finding peace within this final season of Sabbath.

What's needed is healing. That is the balm for the troubled soul, and healing can be found through many methods. What follows are a couple of tools that can bring the healing that opens the door to peace.

The first tool is the Healing Service found in the United Methodist Hymnal and Book of Worship. (The healing service found in other denominations would do the trick, too, but I happen to be a United Methodist pastor.) When the service of healing gets to the laying on of hands and praying, we invoke the Holy

Spirit and ask for healing of body, mind, spirit, and relationships.

The first important word in that prayer is "invoke." We're asking, not demanding, the Holy Spirit to work in our lives. This is the proper attitude since God is not our lackey; we don't get to boss God around. Rather, we are turning to God in a time of need and asking for God's mercy. It is up to God how to respond.

Within that humility is also the notion that God knows better than we do what is needed in that situation. We might be concerned with the failing health of a family member; we want that person to get up and be grandpa again, or to be the good-spirited woman who always hosts the family for Thanksgiving. God, meanwhile, knows that what that person needs most at this hour is acceptance of the situation, or maybe the healing of an estranged relationship. That's why we simply ask for the Holy Spirit to do its thing. We're trusting God's wisdom.

I went into the hospital room of an elderly church member once, and was met by a pastor from another church. He was an old friend of the family, and was just about to wrap up with prayer. I gladly joined in.

While the pastor was praying for this 88-year-old man, he asked God to heal him.

Immediately after saying that, the pastor paused, turned to look at me, and gave a sheepish grin that said he knew that wasn't really the thing to say. After all, what would have been healing for that hospitalized man? Was God going to make him 25 again? Was he going to hop out of bed and do the tango? The healing this man needed had nothing to do with his body. This is why there is such wisdom in any healing service that leaves the decisions up to the Holy Spirit.

Sometimes, though, there will be some healing of the body; just enough to allow some enjoyment of life. This can also go along with a healing of the mind.

There's a common occurrence that happens with patients who have been largely unresponsive or mentally unable to keep up with their surroundings. There will be what the family will call, "a good day." Seemingly out of nowhere, the patient will rally. The family will come in and their loved one is awake, smiling, and knowing exactly who has come to visit. Quite naturally, the family reads this as a sign their loved one has turned the corner and will recover. I've come to conclude this "good day" is an act of grace. God has given enough healing, on a temporary basis, for the family to be able to express their love and say their good-byes. This, in turn, allows for a more peaceful passage. This is the kind of healing that often comes to us from God in the last stage of the Sabbath season.

There's another common occurrence in someone's last days; common enough that it is mentioned in the materials hospice gives the family. This is the phenomena of a dying person seeing people that the rest of us can't see. Typically, these are family members who had passed decades ago.

My father had just entered a new phase. He was aware of people around him, but he could no longer respond coherently to questions. It was as if his mind was on a different plane. While sitting with him in the hospital, not long after he had entered this phase, there was a telling moment. My chair was in a little alcove, tucked out of his line of sight. In addition, the IV pole was between us. To put it simply, I was not in his field of view. Nor was there anyone else in the room. Yet, while I was reading, my wide-awake father distinctly said, "Mom? What are you doing here"?

Such moments are another act of grace. These long-deceased family members remove the fear and anxiety from the mysterious journey we call death. As guides to the next life, they are a comforting presence.

Even with these gifts, the healing of relationships might be the most important healing for finding peace. This was highly visible through Maureen.

Maureen lived alone; just her and her chihuahua. Any hour of the day and night, they could be found sitting together in the living room recliner. Whenever I would visit her, Maureen put on a good face. She was quite entertaining.

However, while talking over things, Maureen would always bring up her youngest daughter, a woman who lived all of three miles away. The problem was that the two women had not spoken to each other in years. This silence came purely from spite. Whatever falling out they'd had, each was too proud to seek a truce, much less reconciliation.

After hashing over the subject, Maureen would inevitably end the discussion by saying, "I don't care if I ever see her again." The falseness of that claim was illustrated by the fact Maureen never failed to mention this painful estrangement with her baby girl. Nothing could have given her greater peace than to have that relationship healed.

You may also have known someone in their last days or hours, who just kept clinging to life until that one person from out of town finally arrived. There was something massively important about seeing that particular person, even if verbal communication was no longer possible.

The importance of relationships leads to another tool that is highly recommended: The Four Things That Matter Most, by Dr. Ira Byock. This simple and easy-to-read book is invaluable for finding peace in relationships as earthly life draws to a close. What follows is a brief discussion of the book's contents but is in no way a substitute for the wisdom in the book itself. I keep copies on hand to give out to people who are facing the death of a family member.

The four things are the four sentences that will ideally be said to each other before a loved one passes over. They tend to represent the things we wish we had said before the opportunity was gone. The first is, "Please forgive me."

Note that it is not, "I'm sorry;" it is, "Please forgive me." That's a request that invites the other person to respond. It asks for engagement. That forgiveness might be communicated through a verbal response, a hug, a squeezing of the hand, or simple tears. Each is a sign of healing.

It's not necessary to go into each and every transgression for which you'd like to apologize. There might be one major incident—the proverbial elephant in the room—that needs to be addressed; but a general, blanket statement will suffice in most cases.

The second sentence is, "I forgive you." Maybe the other person didn't ask. Maybe that person thinks his record is spotless; that she lived a faultless life. That doesn't change the peace you will receive by releasing the grudges you have been clenching for so long. And if that other person does ask, the door has been opened for a beautiful reconciliation, and a lasting peace. That's why, "I forgive you," is a sentence that must be said.

Sentence number three is, "Thank you." What a simple and wonderful way to sum up years of all the necessary and unnecessary kindnesses and acts of caring that mark a relationship. With this sentence you can again sum it up in a few words, as long as the heart is not short-changing the effort. If you feel that deep sense of gratitude, whatever words you say will suffice.

The fourth sentence is the one you've been expecting: "I love you." How often, after an unexpected death due to an accident, a massive stroke, or heart attack, has someone said, "I wish I could have told him I loved him"? Ensure that doesn't happen to you by expressing your love now. You don't have to wait for a terminal illness. Say it now. In fact, say all of the four things now. It is the pathway to healthy relationships, and to the peace that makes the Sabbath season such a joy.

The next tool is to take care of business. If you're reading this because you feel you fit the category, it's time to do all those things listed in the last chapter: put together a will, pre-arrange your funeral, complete an advance directive, and give copies to those who need them.

These are the gifts that are within your power to give your family. But they're also gifts to you. Once you have taken care of these business matters, you can fully embrace the Sabbath season God is giving to you. And it is a season of peace and joy.

When I was recovering from cancer surgery, my big activities for the day were to walk around my neighborhood and to sit on my porch. It was late spring, which meant the trees and sky were full of birds. I loved it. Their songs were captivating. Their activities held my attention. Their colors enlivened what was already beyond gorgeous. Along with the birds, the trees were the color of green you only see in spring, and every yard seemed to have flowers. Because of this, wonder filled each day. That happens every spring, of course, but that year I was open to seeing it. And every scene connected me to the giver of life, the Creator.

This is how each day can be spent during your Sabbath season. These final days are a wonderful time to quiet the self and drink in all God has made. It's a season to be in awe, and to be thankful you've been a part of it. All it requires is an opening of the senses and of the heart.

The other thing that made those neighborhood walks such a joy was stopping and talking to neighbors. Human contact is a gift from the God whose intention was always for us to live in community. During the working years, and even during the active retirement years, life can be so hectic that we rarely spend time with the people living closest to us. We know our co-workers well, we get to know the parents of our children's friends, we'll know the people at church, and as we age we become very familiar with the staff at the doctor's office. Meanwhile, our neighbors get what my own neighbor calls, "the obligatory neighbor wave."

During Sabbath season, we have the time at last to meet the beautiful folks who live next door.

We get to know them. We get to enjoy simple conversation. We get to share recipes and home repair tips. We get to hear the struggles and triumphs of their lives. This is human connection, and it is real; more real than watching the news non-stop. It is what God has always wanted for us. This is what it looks like to live out the command to love our neighbors.

Such encounters bring beauty to each day. They may well be the bright spot. Yet, every day has its moments of beauty. Sabbath season gives us the eyes to see them.

Maybe it's been a rough day. Maybe the day has been filled with pain, setbacks, and disappointments. Such is life. Yet, when your heart is open to the Holy Spirit, you'll notice the grace-filled moments. These could be anything from a welcome phone call, to the smile of a child, to the pill that went down easy for once. Even if there is only one such moment in a given day, it is reason enough to praise God. Such beauty can be found in every single day, and that beauty can redeem the entire 24-hour period.

One more gift of the Sabbath season is reflection of one's life. One of those old tropes is that your life will flash before your eyes in the moment of death, especially when faced with an unexpected life-threatening event. That cliché seems to be one of those things people accept as fact without knowing anyone who's experienced it. What is true without a doubt is that you will have occasion to review your life during eventide. It almost seems to be reflexive. It also tends to be good news.

Among the folks I've attended in their final months, I've heard very little complaining, and very few regrets. There was one woman whose hearing had deserted her during her last decade on earth. It bothered her greatly. Yet, in her final week, she had nothing on her mind but praises to God for the life she'd had.

Such perspective seems to be another gift from our loving Lord. The rough patches are seen nostalgically. The highlights come easier to mind. Even the things that sent us to therapy fade as the joyful moments step to the forefront. In short, the Sabbath season is a time of blissfully thanking God for the experiences, the triumphs, and the joys of your life. This includes the people who shaped you and loved you.

This reflection, along with the other gifts, is what fills our final days with such peace. We're grateful for each new day we spend on earth. We have the peace that comes with appreciating the life we've had, no matter how many years it might have been. We give thanks for healing, and smiles come freely to our lips. All of this leads to the blessed death.

At least among church folks, there's a similarity shared by those who've had a lead-in to their own passing. Whether it was a long illness cutting life short, or the gradual fading at the end of eight or more decades, these folks are ready. Some are tired and desire nothing more than rest, others want to pass over hand-in-hand with those who've come as their guide. Yet, none of them are afraid. In ways we'll only experience when we get there ourselves, they have received assurance from God about what comes next.

Delia was mean, ornery, difficult. It took a lot of stubborn effort to get to know her. She also didn't understand what was going on with her body. She had congestive heart failure, but that term meant nothing to her. She just wanted her next cigarette.

During a visit with her, she shared a dream she'd had. In it, angels had come down from heaven. Saying to her, "Do not fear" these angels took her in their arms and lifted her to heaven. The effect of that dream was immense. Neither of us had any idea Delia would be dead in a month, but she reported that this dream had removed any fear about the rest of her life.

In such mysterious ways, God prepares us for the crossing over. Fear is removed. Peace is bestowed. And if Delia could receive such a gift, there's little doubt you would, too.

Maybe it all comes down to this question: how do you want to exit this world?

There are plenty of ways to do it badly. You can rail at the unfairness of life. You can be consumed by anxiety and fear. You can let them shove a tube down your throat and get your nutrients through yet another tube. You can go out the same way you came in: as a crying, needy, self-centered being.

Or you can live your final years, months, and weeks as a person of faith; someone who trusts deeply in God. When you know you belong to God, there's no fear of death. Instead, you trust the promise of life beyond life; the promise that there is more to come. Because of that sure hope, you can enter into the reward of Sabbath season: a season of peace, joy, and beauty.

Plenty of people choose the former, but perhaps the latter is the narrow road Jesus spoke of in the Sermon on the Mount (Matt. 7:13-14). Maybe the way of faith in our final days is the way that leads not just to life, but to life abundant; a quality of life we have kept at arm's length until now. Through the Holy Spirit, you can change that.

The days are dwindling. The Lord beckons. Choose your road.

AfterLife

"To forget time, to forgive life, to be at peace..."

Oscar Wilde

The Canterbury Ghost

At last we come to an end. Maybe what you've read will make a difference, maybe not. I could be wrong with everything said. Yet, I share from twenty years of experience on the ground as a pastor, plus my own limited experience with illness. This is what I have seen repeatedly.

I've also seen too many people despair as mortality creeps in on them. And it's needless despair. Surely the God who has cared for us all our lives does not abandon us to misery as the sun sets. This book has been a humble attempt to shed light on the alternative approach to our final days and years, a period that can be filled with gratitude and joy.

When we accept that death is not the enemy, but a necessary door to a glorious promise; when we accept that illness and diminished mobility, while not what we desire, are but a new phase of life; when we open ourselves fully to the blessings of the Spirit; resentment and anger depart, and peace comes in like a refreshing rain.

May such peace be yours as you enter your own season of Sabbath.

I come to the end—I am still with you.

Psalm 139:18 (NRSV)

www.ingramcontent.com/pod-product-compliance
Lightning Source LLC
Chambersburg PA
CBHW060258030426
42335CB00014B/1753